21st-CENTURY BAKEMONO:
AN ESSAY ON DIET, CARDIOVASCULAR DISEASES, AND AGING

Author: Dr. Domenico Sarandria, MD

Co-author: Dr. Nicola Sarandria, MD

Dedication by Dr Sarandria Domenico

To my wife, son (and colleague), and my parents.

Copyright 2020

Patamu registry number: 140219

Edited by Scribendi

Dr. Domenico Sarandria:

- Physician, medical doctor; graduated in medicine and surgery from the University of Padova (Italy)
- Specialized in cardiovascular diseases
- Former SICOA Veneto region president
- Chief of Cardiovascular Physiopathology, Villa Torri Hospital, Bologna

Dr. Nicola Sarandria:

- Physician, medical doctor; graduated from Humanitas University (Milan, Italy) in medicine and surgery
- Currently in a Ph.D. position at Humanitas University (Milan, Italy) in molecular and experimental medicine

Table of Contents

Page 1 The cardiovascular system and human health

Page 5 Diet and aging

Page 9 Healthy diets

Page 13 Proper digestion and eating habits

Page 15 The risk of the metabolic syndrome

Page 19 Childhood obesity

Page 21 Changing lifestyles

The cardiovascular system and human health

The cardiovascular system is an intricate apparatus that includes a pump—the heart—and the vasculature, which one can broadly say includes the arteries, veins, and capillaries. As early as the 1600s, Dr. William Harvey first proposed the blood's circulation in the body in his illustrious work *De Motu Cordis* ("the motion of the heart"). Indeed, thanks to this system, we humans are able to function and operate. Moreover, many of the diseases affecting the cardiovascular system are preventable by implementing a correct and healthy lifestyle.

The heart has four chambers, two ventricles, and two atria. It pumps blood throughout the body, which flows through a system of pipes known as *arteries* and *veins*. Microcirculation (which includes the terminal arterioles, metarterioles, venules, and capillaries—along with the lymphatic capillaries) also plays an important role. It serves mainly to deliver oxygen and nutrients, remove carbon dioxide, and regulate inflammation as well as edema formation.

In the arteries, an abnormal accumulation of macrophages, lipids, debris, calcium, and fibrous connective tissue can occur. This accumulation is called *atheromatous plaque*. It can occlude various arteries at different levels (a decrease in the lumen is known as *stenosis*). If a critical stenosis occurs in the coronary system, it could complicate into a myocardial infarction—a heart attack.

Cholesterol-panel levels, including low-density lipoproteins (LDL), predict cardiovascular, diseases such as ischemic coronary syndromes. Various molecules have been implemented as a medical therapy to reduce cholesterol levels, including statins (HMG-CoA inhibitors), ezetimibe (which affects intestinal absorption), and novel monoclonal antibodies, such as evolocumab (which blocks the hepatic protein called *PCSK9* from interfering with the binding of LDL to these superficial liver proteins).

Interestingly, Omega-3 oil (which is contained, for instance, in fish and nuts and is, therefore, available both from animal and vegetal origins) has been shown to reduce triglycerides levels, therefore aiding in the prevention of atheromatous plaques. Also, the isomer trans-resveratrol—which is contained in grape seeds, for instance—has been shown to help reduce the risk of a cardiovascular event and act on the sirtuin group of genes (e.g., Sirt 7), thus counteracting some physio-pathological effects of aging. These examples emphasize lifestyles' massive impact on cardiovascular disease, showing how diet can affect the body at a genetic level. Diet can provide a stronger base upon which lay the foundations of the "healthy diet" concept.

Diet and aging

With the advent of new technologies, we found ourselves able to live longer lives. Quality of life has never been so important, and diet is a cornerstone of healthy living.

When discussing diet and its impact on aging, first considering aging as a multifactorial process that the human body undergoes is essential. Aging involves various processes. Inflammation, for example, is a multifaceted process that can be acute, sub-acute, or chronic, It is vital for the human body to survive and fight off diseases or infections; however, it can also be detrimental and cause disease. Indeed, silent, chronic inflammation is a leading cause of disease, and it often accompanies aging. The chronic inflammation process is correlated with several pathologies, such as stroke, myocardial infarction, neurological disease, and oncological disease. The triggers of this type of inflammation include lifestyle and diet.

Glycation is another major point in discussing the aging process, cardiovascular diseases, and diet. It is a biochemical reaction that depends on the presence and concentration of glucose in the blood, of proteins, and of cells' permeability to glucose. The results of this process are glycotoxins, which alter the tissues and induce AGE (advanced glycation end-products), causing inflammation and ROS (reactive oxidative species)–producing processes.

Also worth mentioning is DNA methylation, which is a physiological process necessary for the formation and reparation of DNA and, in some types of genes, silencing processes where genes get inactivated. DNA methylation is involved in the production of various macromolecules, such as lipids, neurotransmitters, proteins, hormones, and nerves' myelin sheaths. However, when this process changes—in turn, affecting the epigenetic landscape of human DNA—it can have a detrimental effect on the human body. For instance, a downstream effect of an altered methylation process is an increase in homocysteine levels, which increases the risk of cardiovascular diseases, such as stroke. (Homocysteine is considered an independent risk factor for atherosclerosis, and it has been shown to induce an inflammatory response in vascular, smooth muscle cells (Pang X et al., 2014).

Another factor related to ageing-causing processes is Oxidative stress can induce an increase in ROS production, both from endogenous causes (such as obesity or diabetes mellitus) and exogenous causes (like alcohol, smoke or pesticides).

In relation to oxidative stress and stress imposed on human bodies, there are means to quantitatively and qualitatively measure it. For instance, quantitative blood cortisol levels could offer an effective means in certain categories of the population (like in certain groups of patients affected by psychological stressors), together with its axis (ACTH). DHEA (Dehydroepiandrosterone) and sex hormones, together with urinary catecholamines and glycemic, could also be effective serological markers for stress. Basal and under-stimulus biofeedback is a further method to measure stress. This feedback measures galvanic resistance on the skin (by measuring electric currents on the skin of the patient).

Healthy diets

Diet is fundamental for a correct and balanced lifestyle. For instance, processed meat, nitrite-rich foods (together with other cancerogenic preservers), lead-rich vegetables, and burnt food (which can be rich in some instances of acrylamide—a cancerogenic substance) can have negative health effects. Therefore, certain foods are deleterious and—in some instances, if chronically consumed—could lead to serious pathologies (such as caners and cardiovascular diseases). As we saw in the previous section "The cardiovascular system and human health," diet and cardiovascular diseases (CVD) are intricately connected. One of the most important effects in this connection is diet and cholesterol, which share a strong and long-established relationship.

A healthy diet must necessarily contain the five main food groups.

1) Vegetables and legumes

2) Fruits

3) Grains (cereals)

4) Lean meats, poultry, fish, and eggs

5) Milk, yogurt, Cheese, or alternatives (mostly with reduced fat content)

Moreover, preparing food with healthy cooking methods (for instance cooking using water vapour) can strongly affect the properties of the foods we consume. Lipids—preferably, rich in unsaturated fats and low in saturated fats—should also be included. White meats and fish are also part of a healthy diet, but when eating meat, the animals ought to have lived and grown in the open, fed on grass, and been spared the heavy use of antibiotics. These aspects of a healthy diet also allow for better control of cholesterol levels, helping to prevent atherosclerosis.

It is important to categorize foods as "functional foods," with clear benefits to our bodies. These functional foods include "superfoods" (nutritionally dense foods) like green tea and garlic. These foods were commonly used in various cultures and past rural populations, showing superfoods' amazing benefits and highlighting the need to return to a more rural lifestyle, including physical activity and a healthier diet. Removing fast foods and processed foods and focusing instead on raw, organic materials can help us cook in healthy ways.

Another important aspect of considering a healthy diet, too often forgotten, is the use of pesticides in our food.

Trying to eat organic food helps ensure the healthy benefits of the products we eat daily.

Regarding condiments, salt monitoring is a necessary observation in our everyday lives. It should consider not only the salt we add to meals ourselves but also the existing salt contained in many of the pre-made foods we buy.

Proper digestion and eating habits

Digestion starts in the mouth. Importantly, we must remind ourselves to chew our foods 15 to 30 times so that the enzymes in our saliva, and the mechanical grinding of our teeth, can start the proper digestion process.

As we saw in the previous section, it is also important to cut back on restaurants and take-out meals as much as possible. Restaurants and take-out foods are often rich in salts, preservatives, trans-saturated fats, and refined sugars—all of which are detrimental to both cardiovascular health and our bodies' overall physiology.

An important tip to keep in mind is, "Eat like a king in the morning." The morning is when you need energy and nutrients to face the day ahead. Eating a balanced and nutrient-filled lunch will sustain you for the remainder of the day and keep your body going. Finally, eat a very light dinner. Be sure not to eat dinner too late. Enjoying the day's final meal at around 6:00 PM allows your body to digest before going to bed light—which will also help prevent gastroesophageal reflux GERD).

The risk of the metabolic syndrome

Foods and drinks like soft drinks, sodas, and confectionaries are often high in glycemic value and calories. They might lead to overweight and obesity, which is a true epidemic in many countries that causes terrifying effects on the human body (such as diabetes mellitus type II, hypertension, heart attack, cancer). As humans, we have collectively forgotten how an excessive intake of food—combined with the astounding decrease in physical activity that has, unfortunately, been recorded in many countries around the globe—can have destructive and perhaps highly preventable effects.

Overweight and obesity lead to metabolic syndrome. And, if there were ever an important time to talk about this syndrome, it is now. When we physicians refer to *metabolic syndrome*, we use this medical term to describe the combination of diabetes mellitus, hypertension (high arterial blood pressure), and obesity. This syndrome puts sufferers at a much higher risk of cardiovascular diseases, such as coronary artery disease (an increased risk of myocardial Infarction—heart attack) and stroke. These conditions included in metabolic syndrome are, indeed, often linked. Data from the NHS in the United Kingdom have shown that these conditions affect one in three adults over 50 years old in the United Kingdom.

Symptoms of metabolic syndrome include:

- High blood triglyceride levels and low HDL levels (a risk factor for atherosclerosis)
- High arterial blood pressure (often 140/90 mmHg)
- A waist circumference above 94 cm for men and 80 cm for women (European populations)

- An inability to control blood sugar levels (signs of insulin resistance, an alarm bell for the development of diabetes mellitus Type II)

- An increased risk of developing blood clots (e.g., deep vein thrombosis—DVT)

- Increased inflammation

The causes of metabolic syndrome include being overweight or obese (with a lack of exercise), age, insulin resistance, and the presence of diseases (such as non-alcoholic liver disease, polycystic ovary syndrome, and cardiovascular diseases). So, preventing or reversing metabolic syndrome possible? The answer is yes!

The key to preventing or reversing metabolic includes mostly lifestyle changes, such as increasing isotonic physical exercise, eating a healthy diet (low in salt, low in saturated fats, and low in refined sugars), quitting smoking, and quitting drinking alcoholic beverages. Also, under the counsel of your personal physician, medical therapy can be implemented.

We live in a very different society than our ancestors. Food is more accessible, and the advent of cheap and worldwide distribution has made fast-food ailments widespread. Most families on the different continents consume fast food. This change has especially affected young generations, leading to the next topic in this essay: childhood obesity. This issue has become one of the most serious public health threats of this century.

Childhood obesity

The prevalence of obesity (and overweight) among adolescents is classified according to the World Health Organization growth reference for school-aged children and adolescents (namely, 2 and 1 standard deviations in body mass index or BMI, by sex and age, for obesity and overweight, respectively). This issue is ever-increasing, and it affects many low- and high-income countries. In 2016, the number of overweight children under the age of five was estimated at 41 million. These children are more likely to remain overweight or obese during their adult lives, leading to a plethora of preventable conditions, such as cardiovascular diseases and diabetes mellitus Type II, at a very young age.

Also importantly, approximately 2.5 million people die yearly due to overweight and obesity complications.

These individuals are not only at higher risk of developing certain types of cancers (such as endometrial, breast, and colon cancer) but also osteoarthritis.

Our societies have undergone a clear shift to very energy-rich diets, filled with saturated fats, refined sugars, and salt. This change, together with a marked decrease in physical activity, has led to a veritable pandemic that is affecting future generations and remodeling society itself —including the public health in various countries. Even more than adults, children need specialized attention to fight obesity and overweight. These interventions also involve teaching about the short-term and long-term consequences of this type of lifestyle.

Changing lifestyles

As we are near the conclusion of this essay, a final concept is worth noting. Despite the last decades' reduction in age-adjusted mortality, in 2013, cardiovascular disease (CVD) was the leading cause of death in the United States (indeed, CVDs have been a leading cause of death in the United States for the last hundred years). These cardiovascular diseases include coronary artery diseases (the most common), cerebrovascular diseases (strokes), peripheral arteries diseases, and many other conditions under this umbrella term.

It is very important to note that many conditions included in the term *cardiovascular diseases* are preventable, which brings us to the primary and secondary prevention methods of Cardiovascular diseases. In primary prevention, importantly, the target patient group has no cardiovascular diseases, and the aim is preventing the onset of these conditions. Secondary-prevention measures target patients with cardiovascular diseases, aiming to prevent the onset of new CVDs and the worsening of pre-existing conditions. Both preventions deal with the plethora of aspects and "weapons" in the medical community's arsenal to fight this devastating public health burden. These interventions include lifestyle changes and medications (such as treating hypertension, and also multi-drug regimens and treating dyslipidemia).

Our lifestyles deeply affect our genetic background, life expectancy, and quality of life. Let's make the best of them!

www.ingramcontent.com/pod-product-compliance
Lightning Source LLC
Chambersburg PA
CBHW070914220526
45466CB00005B/2208